ACCENT AFRICAN

Traditional
and
Contemporary
Hairstyles
for the
Black Woman

THIRD EDITION

Text by
Valerie Thomas-Osborne
and
Carla Brown

Hairstyles by
Carla Brown
Sonia Bullock
James Finney
Elizabeth Fripp
Nicol Missette
Donna Moses
Isoke Niyalínghi

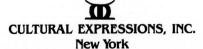

CULTURAL EXPRESSIONS, INC.
New York

D1292712

ISBN: 0-9629827-0-9

CREDITS

Editor *Dr. Columbus Salley.*
Cover Photos *Joe Harris,* top row. *Gene Ward,* bottom row.
Cover Hairstyles *Carla Brown* African Twists (top row, left), cornrows (bottom row, left), Individual Twists (bottom row, left). *Elizabeth Fripp* Medium Individuals (top row, right).
Cover Makeup *Nzingha Gumbs* (top row, left).
Text Photos *Joe Harris* pages 9, 18, 19, 20, 21, 22, 23, 32, (left), 33 (left), 45, 53, 56, 57, and 65. *Bob Gumbs* pages 10, 11, 14, 15, 16, 17, 26, 27, 30, 31, 34, 38, 39, 46, 48, 49, 50, 54, 58, 60 and 61. *Kwame Brathwaite* page 12, 13, 24, 25, 28, 35, 42, 43, 52 and 59. *Gene Ward* pages 29, 32 (right), 33 (right), 36 (left), 40 (right), 41 (left), 44 (left). *Perry Williams* pages 36 (right), 37, 40 (left), 41 (right), 44 (right) and 66. *Richard Sookradge* pages 62, 63 and 64.
Text Photos Makeup *Nzingha Gumbs* pages 9, 18, 19, 20, 21, 32 (left), 33 (left), 34, 45, 56, and 65. *Sajada Robinson* pages 12, 13, 24, 25, 28, 42, 43, 52 and 53.
Text Illustrations *Yvette Jenkins.*

Book Design *Bob Gumbs.*

Contents

Introduction

Since the first edition of *ACCENT AFRICAN: Traditional and Contemporary Hairstyles for the Black Woman* was published in 1973, the African art of cornrowing and braiding has become a popular expression of cultural identity for Black women.

The history of cornrowing and braiding can be traced to Africa as far back as 3500 B.C. Sculptured hairstyles played an important role in the daily lives of African people — defining one's age and status in the community.

Throughout the centuries, cornrowing and braiding continued to have political, social, cosmetic, holistic and cultural significance.

Today, because of the increased demand for African hairstyles, beauty and hair salons have added professional African hairstylists to their staffs. A growing number of hair salons are specializing in African hairstyling exclusively.

This ancient African art form is also becoming more accepted in the field of cosmetology and beauty schools are including African hairstyling in their curriculum. Further, hair magazines regularly feature African hairstyles.

The third edition of *ACCENT AFRICAN* contains over 72 Cornrows, Braids, Locs, Interlocs, African Twists, Nubian Twists and Corkscrew styles. Because over the years African hairstyles have become popular with Black men, for the first time, *ACCENT AFRICAN* has included a number of these styles. We also have expanded our selection of hairstyles for children.

Once again, we invite you to experience the art and beauty of African hairstyling.

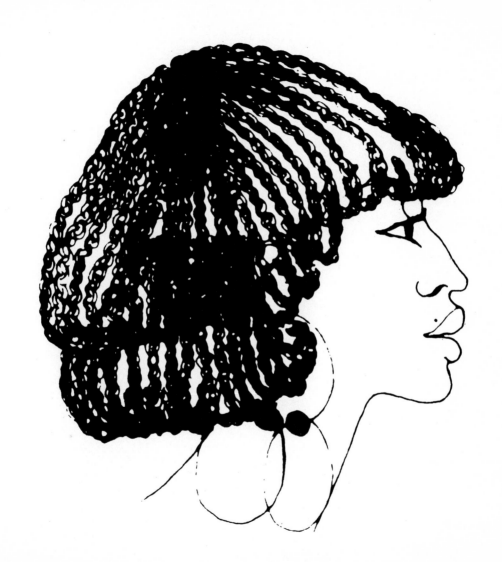

The Art of Cornrowing

Cornrowing is an ancient art handed down from generation to generation in Africa. It is representative of the symmetry and order of African Womens' beauty habits; in essence, it is an expression of communion with the universe.

Cornrowing is a basic aesthetic of the African woman's existence. It is considered the living art form of millions of women from West, South, East and Central Africa. There are countless variations of it and no one style appears the same way on any one woman. For example, in Nigeria cornrowing is looked upon as an art akin to spirituality and ritual. Traditionally, among the Yoruba, the most decorative and intricate styles were worn by priestesses and queens. Not only was cornrowing a symbol of status during these times, but was also a sign of age. Young girls and older women wore simple, basic styles, while marriagable women wore the more elaborate versions.

Today's Black American women, with their new pride and dignity, can also experience the spirituality, grace, and beauty of the art of cornrowing.

STEP 1 To begin simply oil and brush your hair. Then part the hair into 3 sections, as if you were going to braid a pigtail. Take care to hold only a minimum amount of hair at a time and begin to interweave sections.

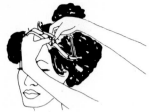

Interweave section 3 over section 2.
Then part the lower portion of 3.

STEP 2 This must be done similtaneously while plucking hair from the roots and weaving it into each section. All cornrowing must be done flat on the surface of the scalp. When you reach the end of the hair, simply twist or braid this hair.

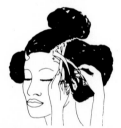

Join sections 3 and 4 under section 1.
(Section 1 should be in the middle over sections 3 and 4.)

STEP 3 Keeping the cornrow in harmony with the parted scalp is essential to the success of any cornrow style. Cornrows should be tight and may feel excessively tight your first time, but the tighter the better. Thickness depends upon your own individual hair, as does the amount of time involved. It is possible to spend 45 minutes or 3 hours or more cornrowing.

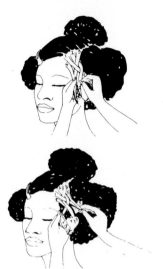

Join section 5 with section 2.
Twist sections 2, 3, and 4 around section 1.

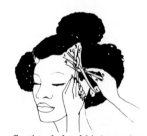

Section 1 should join section 6.
(All sections should now be interwoven.)

Now that you have finished cornrowing, you are ready to begin experimenting with the countless hair styles available to beautiful Black women.

How to Add Extensions

If you have short or thin hair and would like to wear one of the longer braided styles, this may be done by adding synthetic or human hair pieces (extensions).

To begin, detach several small sections from your hairpiece and lay them close at hand.

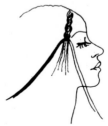

STEP 1 Evenly part a section of your own hair and

either at the beginning of your braid or midway into the braid, lay the extension over the natural hair. The center of the extension should meet the natural hair section.

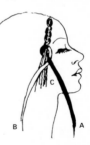

STEP 2 Start to braid, passing section A under section C and over section B.

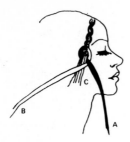

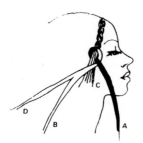

STEP 3 Pass section B over section C. The extension should now be securely in place.

STEP 4 Pull some hair from section B, forming section D and blend into natural hair (section C). Then complete your braid.

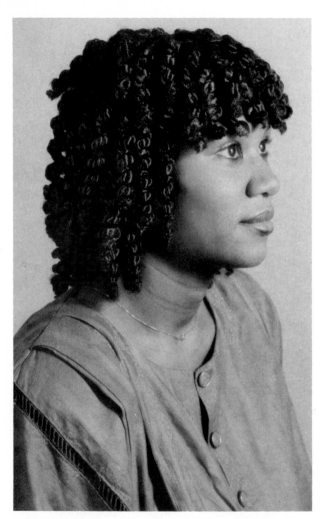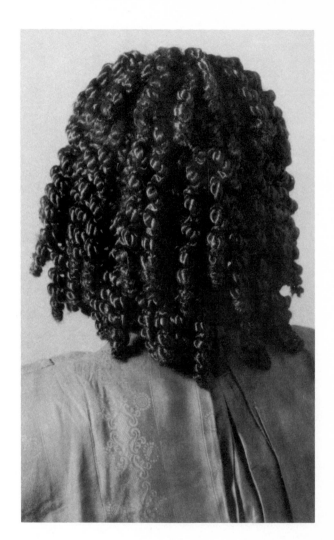

African Twist Layers. *Hairstyle by Carla Brown.*

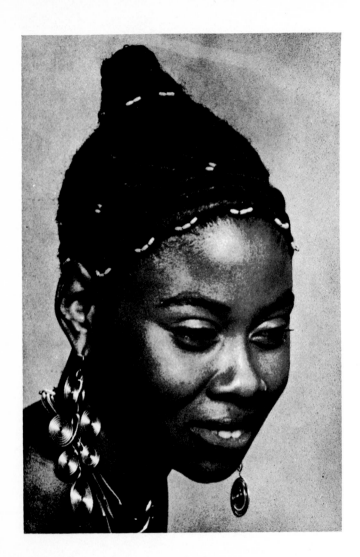

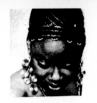

Adama *by Sonia Bullock*

The Adama (Queenly) is similar to a traditional West African style. It works best on women with short to medium length hair. While styling takes between 2 and 2½ hours, the Adama results are well worth the time.

Before beginning to style the hair, make sure you have a comb, brush, bobby pins and rubber bands. Note: if the hair is short to medium, a long braided piece will be necessary.

Begin by brushing the hair. Then comb the hair in an upward fashion. Start parting at the nape of the neck. These parts should be very thin, along the hair line; they should also create a complete circle around the head. (This will form the first row of cornrows.) Continue this procedure for two more rows. All cornrows should be small.

When this is completed, comb out hair and find the center of the head. From this point begin to part in a swirl effect (see photo), going to the top of the head. Continue this all the way around the head, keeping in mind that the curve must be followed for favorable results.

After this is done, band the cornrows at the top; flip them over and pin them so that they are not standing up.

Now you are ready to add the braid. This is done by pinning the braid to the scalp. Be certain that the braid is secure.

Then begin to wrap the braid around the exposed hair at the top. Tuck this hair under the braid and pin down.

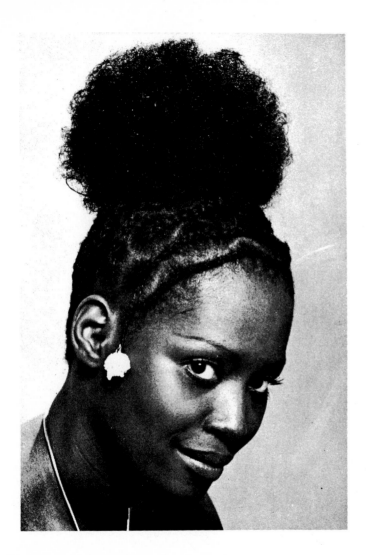

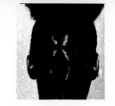

Aissatou *by Sonia Bullock*

The Aissatou is a universal hairstyle. To style the Aissatou, comb the hair in an upward direction. Part the hair from the ear to the top of the forehead, along the hair line. This part should be scalloped. Now begin to cornrow from right to left—allowing this cornrow to hang loosely.

Switch now to the left ear, parting in the scalloped effect over the right ear. This effect will cause the two parts to form a figure 8 design (see photo).

Begin to braid a second cornrow in the opposite direction (leave this hanging loosely).

At the center of the head, part the top into 4 sections. Tie off 3 of these and, with the 1 remaining section, begin to part with the scalloped effect once more. *Be sure that loose hairs are clipped down.*

Now part the other side of the cornrow, so that the scallops are now facing away from each other. The scallop parts should start where the cornrows end.

Begin to cornrow from the front of the head to the top. Take each of the other pinned sections out and follow this same pattern.

Remember that the angles of the hair should be from the nape of the neck straight up to the top to create the back; from the ear straight up to the top of the head, creating the sides (scallops get smaller the nearer they are to the top).

When all cornrows reach the top, band them together and comb them out. This creates a puff effect.

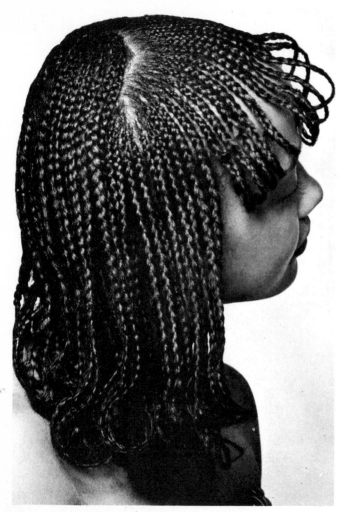
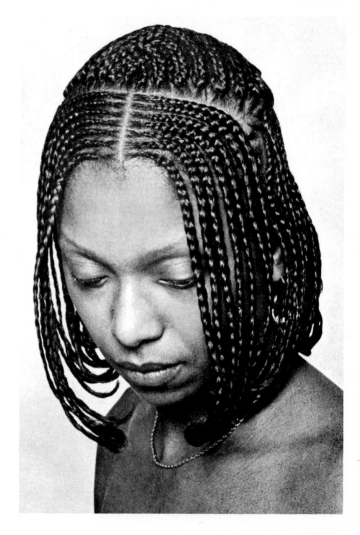

Hairstyles by Donna Moses

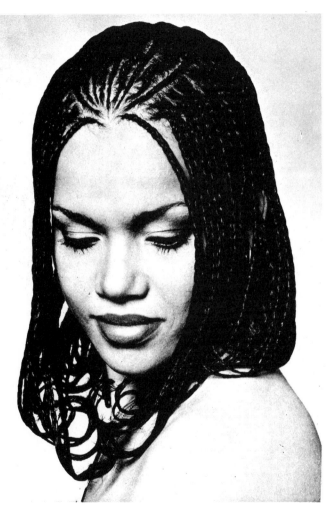

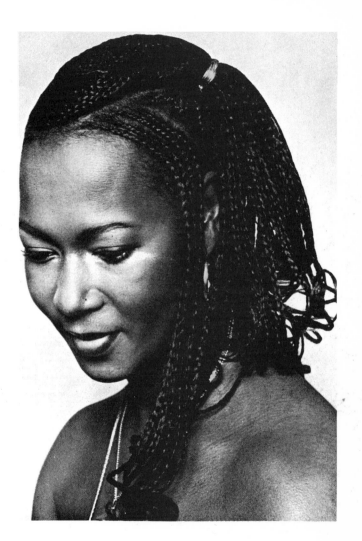

Hairstyles by Donna Moses

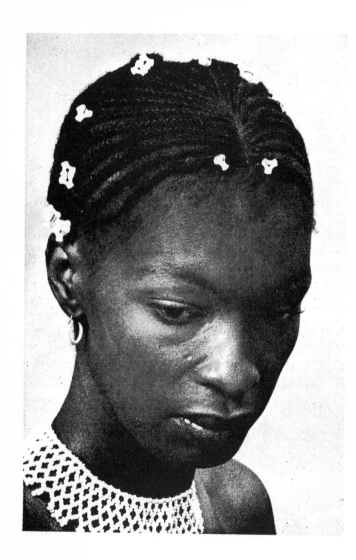

NZinga *by Sonia Bullock*

Yorubaland has inspired the NZinga, (pronounced N-Zinga). Most of the time, Yoruban women wear their hair wrapped, but when it is not, it appears in a style somewhat like the NZinga. For this style, the hair must be medium length, not too short or too long.

To begin, part the hair into two sections across the top of the head, from ear to ear. The back section should be tied off for now. Part in front, up the center half way towards the top. Comb the hair to the side. Pin the left side down.

First, cornrow from the top center to the side part, along the hair line. Do the same for 5 or more cornrows.

For the top, start at the center going to the top of the head. This should be done on an angle to create a starburst effect. Take the other side (left) out and repeat these steps. Pin the braids back so that they will not be in the way.

The back is done the same as the front. Once this is completed, connect the braids from the center to the end and wrap them around the ear (see photo).

Although the NZinga is an everyday hairstyle, adornments do make an attractive difference.

14

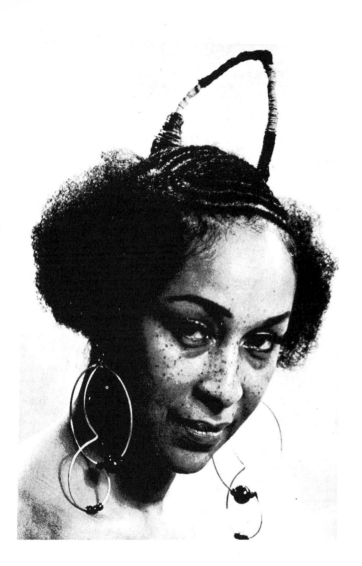

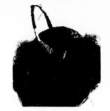

Monifa *by Sonia Bullock*

The Monifa is very similar to an Ethiopian mode of hairstyling. It suits ladies with medium length, kinky or fine grade hair. It suits formal wear best.

Before you begin to work with the hair, make sure you have hair clips, pick, comb, threads, and a hair piece (braid).

When you are ready, start by parting the hair into 3 sections. The first section should be parted from the temple down to the back. This part should not go straight down to the back, but should stop slightly above the base of the neck.

Do the same thing on the opposite side of the head. These are the two outer sections. Tie both of these off and work with the remaining hair.

Start now at the top of the head. Part this hair in half; this creates a part going across the top of the head. Place clips in the hair to hold the back section down; toward the front of this, begin braiding small cornrows. Do the same with the back part of this section.

Wrap the back of the hair about a half inch deep with colored thread, 4 strands thick.

Make or use a thin braid for the top portion of this section. Lay the braid on the cornrow and wrap it around the hair, changing threads colors. Then attach the piece to one of the braids in front. When you reach the end of the hair, tie the threads, making a knot.

The sides and the back should be combed, brushed and picked; then pat into shape.

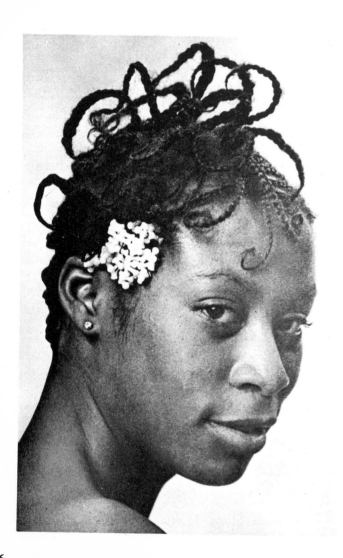

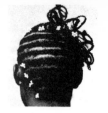

Billie Holiday *by Sonia Bullock*

The Billie Holiday is truly a Black American creation, inspired by Lady Day herself. It is most suitable for medium to long hair. The grooming aids needed include: comb, brush, clips and beads.

The Billie Holiday is essentially a 3 section hairdo. The first section begins with a part from the left side at the temple, around in a circle to the right side, stopping just over the ear (all of this hair is considered one section).

The top part of this section should be the beginning of a long cornrow, following the established part. At the bottom, begin to braid from left to right. When you reach the right side, the cornrow should end directly over the ear. This should be left hanging loosely. Continue the same step all the way around.

You should now have several loose braids on the right side. Adjoin these from the nape of the neck to the area just above the ear. This completes the bottom portion.

Comb the hair out on the top section (section two) and begin parting it from the brow on the right side to the top of the head. Pin down the right side for now.

Cornrow from the edge of the hair up to the part, from left to right. Braid horizontally across the head, also from left to right. Do this all the way around, leaving the braids to hang loosely.

Now take out the last section (three) and make a small series of box braids. Roll these braids up on the right side with curlers (*do not use hot curlers*). Remove them and pat the Billie Holiday into shape.

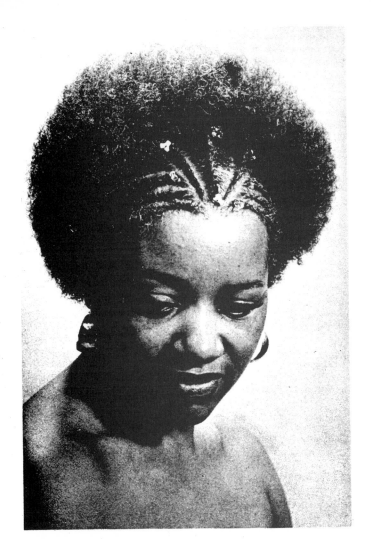

Wisdom's Crown *by Sonia Bullock*

Another variation of the traditional Ethiopian style is Wisdom's Crown. To create the style, bobby pins, a comb, brush and, perhaps, a hair piece should be within reach.

Once again, cornrowing is essential. Begin by parting the hair for a large cornrow to be made around the head. The remaining hair should be pulled back for braiding.

Complete a circle of cornrows (any number desired, so long as there is ample hair for picking out). Now take the remaining hair out, part once again. (By now you should be at the crown of the head.) Section off four more cornrows, creating one large cornrow at the top.

Take out the sectioned off hair; comb and pick. You may now pat hair into the desired shape.

For height, a hair piece may be attached or a small hat or crown.

Wisdom's Crown looks best when worn with closed neck attire rather than jewelry; likewise, a rounded neckline adds to the effect. Small earrings may be added for simple adornment.

This is essentially a casual, everyday hair style and is not intended for dressy occassions.

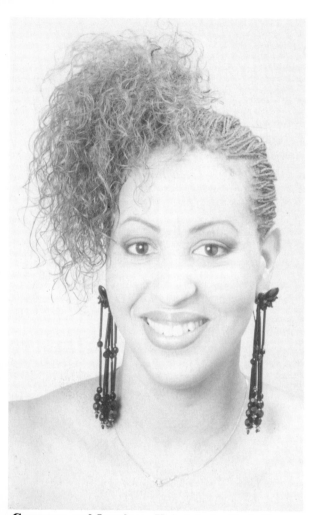

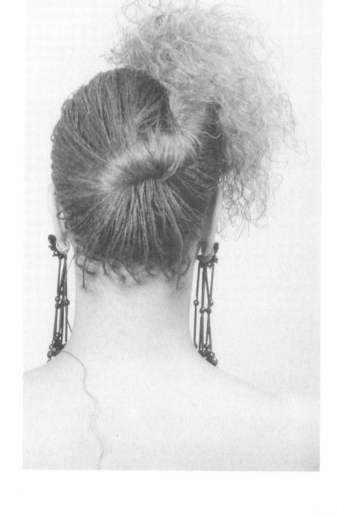

Cornrows and Interlocs. *Hairstyle by Carla Brown.*

18

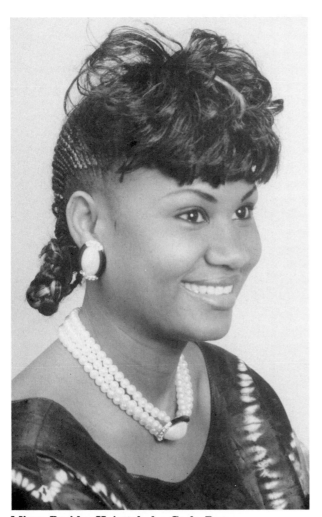 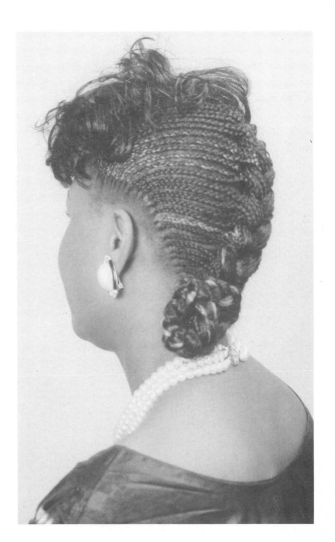

Micro Braids. *Hairstyle by Carla Brown.*

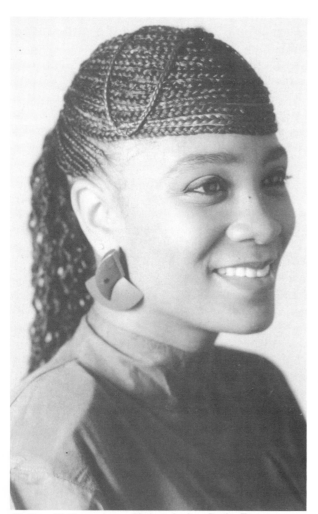
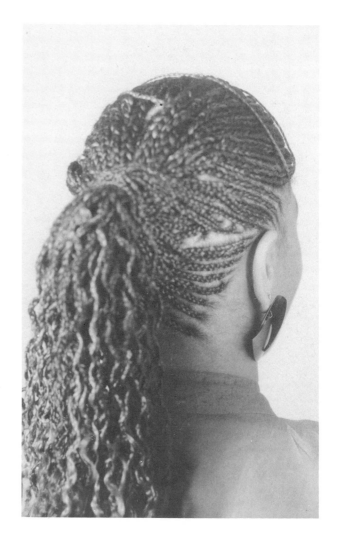

Kofe, all Cornrows. *Hairstyle by Carla Brown.*

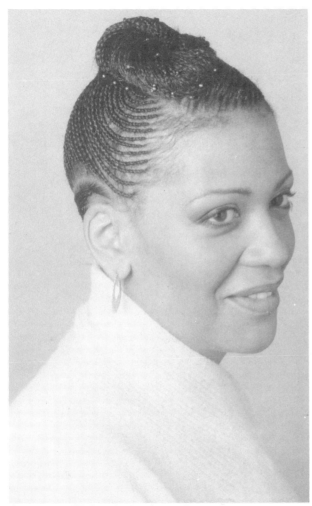

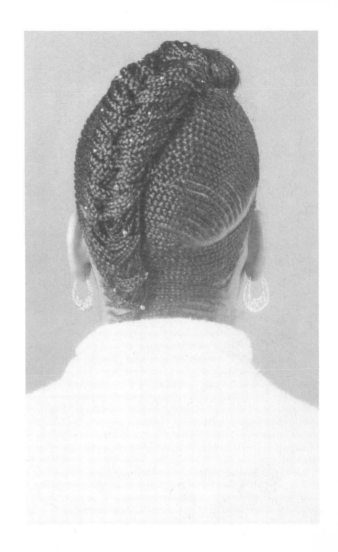

Cornrows. *Hairstyle by Carla Brown.*

21

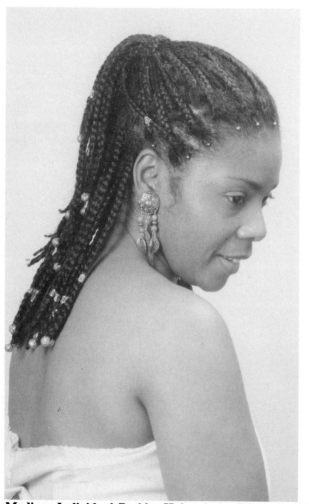
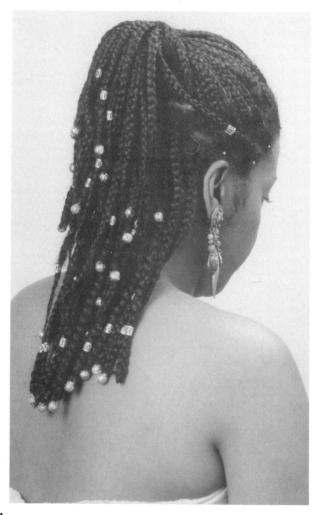

Medium Individual Braids. *Hairstyle by Elizabeth Fripp.*

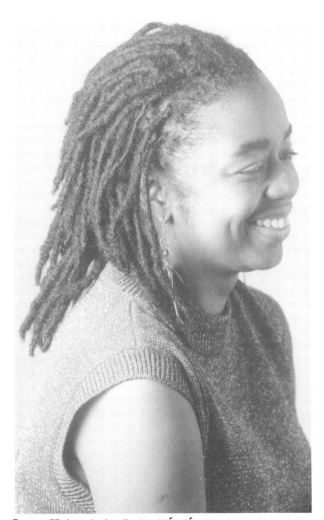
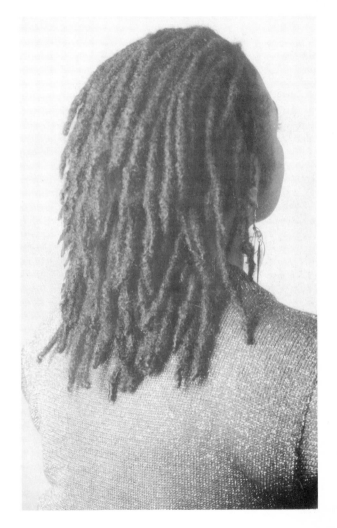

Locs. *Hairstyle by Isoke Níyalínghi.*

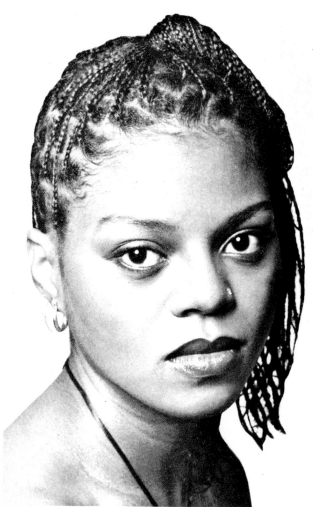

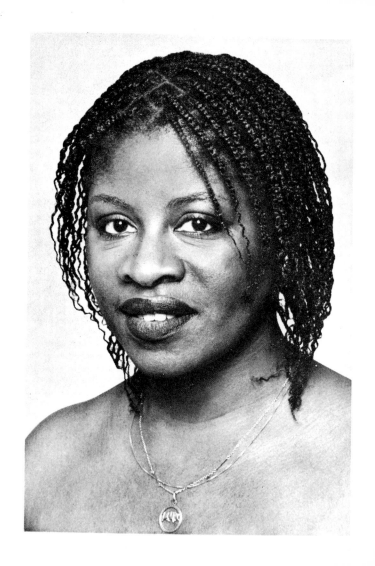

Fplaits by James Finney

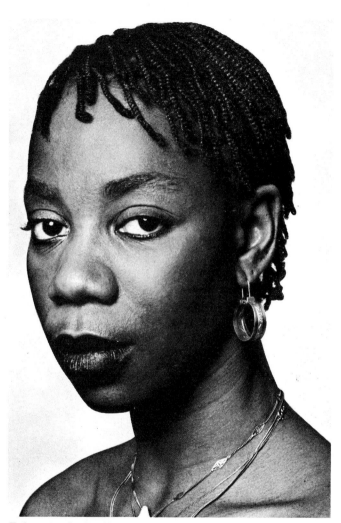

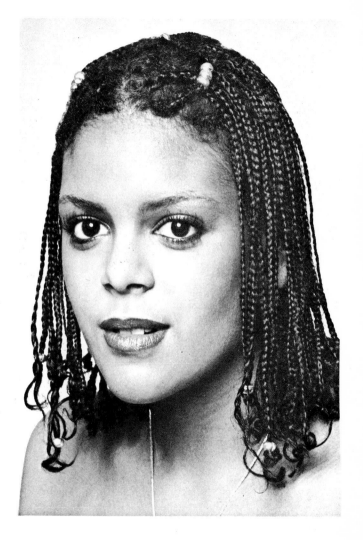

Fplaits by James Finney

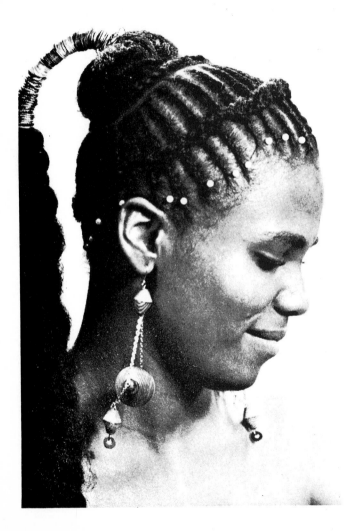

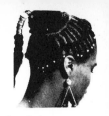

Ayanna *by Sonia Bullock*

Ayanna means beautiful flower in Yoruba. It is most ideal for women with long, thick hair. Have on hand a comb, brush, bobby pins, rubber bands and string.

Divide the hair into 3 equal sections. Begin with a part around the center of the top of the head. This should be round shaped. Band together loose hair with rubber bands. Next, section the hair off.

Section 1. Part down the center and comb the hair to sides. Pin the left side down. The right side begins with small, tight braids, from the hairline to the part. Continue to center-back. Do the same on the other side. Braiding the braids all the way to the end.

Section 2. Braid from the top to the front with small braids parallel with sections all the way around to the center back. Repeat on the other side.

Starting at the center back (left side), connect the braids by interlocking (weaving braids together), all the way around to the right side center-back.

Section 3. Remove the rubber band, then comb and brush. About two inches of the hair should be wrapped with thread. Let one inch of hair hang loose and continue to wrap at the end of the inch going down (this depends on length). Leave a pony tail hanging at the end. This may be achieved by using a hairpiece.

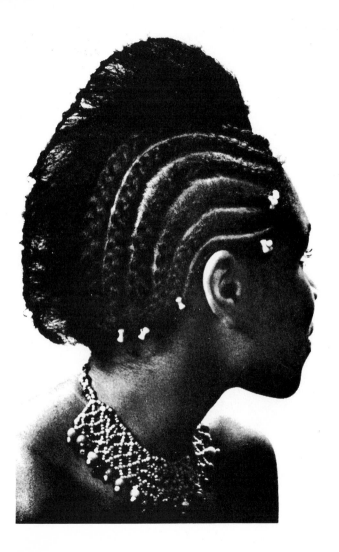

Angel's Arch *by Sonia Bullock*

The Peul women of Upper Volta (near Ghana) often wear their hair twisted and combed into a fan effect at the center of the head. A more contemporary version of this hairstyle is the Angel's Arch.

This style is most suitable for women with fairly long, evenly cut hair. Before beginning to style, wash and condition hair; prepare to use comb, brush, bobby pins, and a hair conditioner.

To begin, part hair from front to back—from the temple to right behind the ear. Section off the hair and pin it with bobby pins.

Starting from the hairline (temple), cornrow back to behind the ear. Make these thick and large. Make another cornrow of the same length right next to this one. Both of these should be going around the head in its natural shape. The third cornrow starts at the center of the hairline (forehead), and goes around the head, as the previous two.

In order to create the fan effect for the center, hair should be combed straight up and then brushed straight out, along the shape of the head. Now with the palms of your hands, take the hair and squeeze it together.

Proceed to cornrow, pulling on the ends of the hair in an upward motion, connecting them as you cornrow. The connecting is done best by taking small pieces of hair at a time. All of this should be done down the center of the head. The part should be the same width as the cornrow.

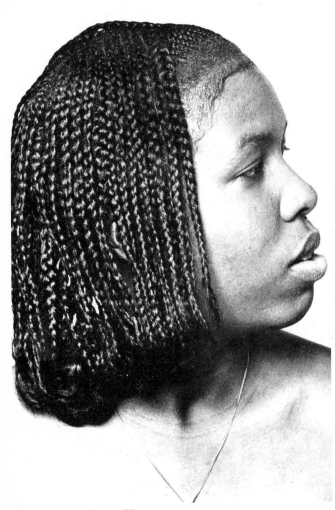
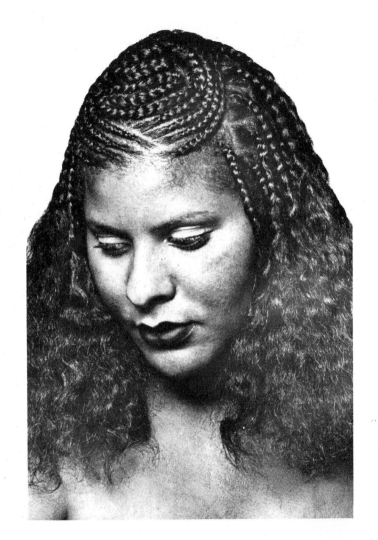

Hairstyles by Donna Moses

28

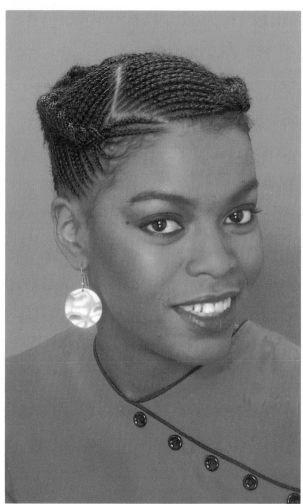
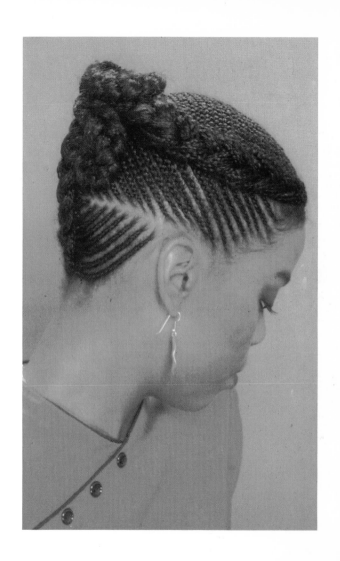

Cornrows and Extensions.
Hairstyle by Carla Brown.

29

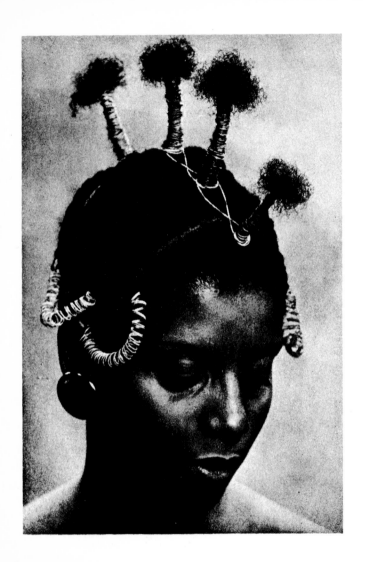

Twana *by Sonia Bullock*

Twana is based on an African hair style commonly called "Trees".

This style is most popular in West and Central Africa.

Twana means alive; and this style allows for breadth and comfort.

The hair should be fair textured, medium-to-short in length. A small faced woman would look best in this casual style.

Have a comb, brush, rubber bands and thread available.

Start by parting the hair into 5 sections. Part from ear to ear acorss the front. Part again from ear to ear across the top of the head. Make sure that you have the same amount of hair in each section.

The other sections include from ear-to-ear across the upper back of the head, ear-to-ear across the middle back, and ear-to-ear across bottom back. Section these off with rubber bands.

Proceed to cornrow each section, and wrap each center section with thread, wrapping ¾ of the entire hair's length. Do the same with each section. Comb out the top of the hair and pat into shape. Different color threads may be used.

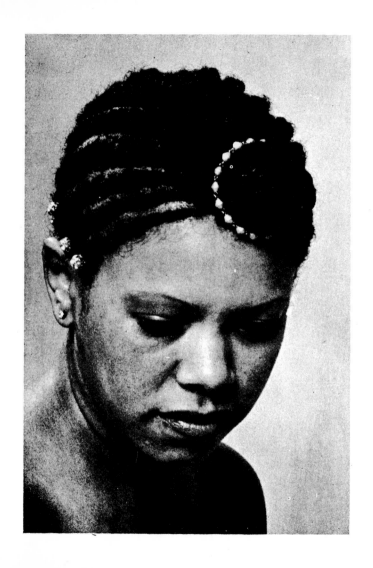

Shalewa *by Sonia Bullock*

The Shalewa style is simple in appearance. It should be worn casually and without much decoration. It can be worn by any age woman, with any length of hair.

First part the hair at the top frontal area of head. This area should be about 2 inches from the hairline. This hairstyle involves a sunburst effect, so you should part outward. Next, from the temple begin to twist tightly the hair at the very edges (of the hairline), all the way to the back. This should be done on both sides of the head.

Now, part hair at the center of the head and make one medium width cornrow beginning at the base of head up to the top; to accompany this cornrow, make a series of braids all equaling the width of the cornrow. Make sure that these braids part into squares.

By this time you should have one large cornrow going up the center of the head to the part, with a series of braids on each side of it.

Now from the top of the ear part upwards. Begin french rolling (this is cornrowing in reverse see page 29), to the "front center" of head.

From the center of the ear, part again (this time on a curve) and braid a series of small braids in squares.

Next, cornrow and frenchrow a series of braids. These should all meet the large cornrow in the center. This will form the back.

Lastly, pull the hairs at the top together and tie into a loop or a knot.

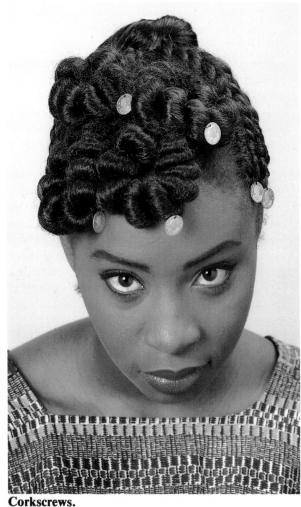

Corkscrews.
Hairstyle by Carla Brown.

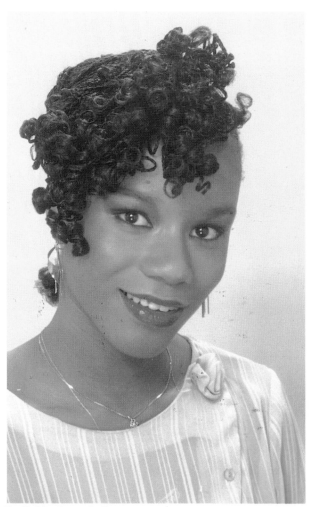

Individuals and Cornrows.
Hairstyle by Carla Brown.

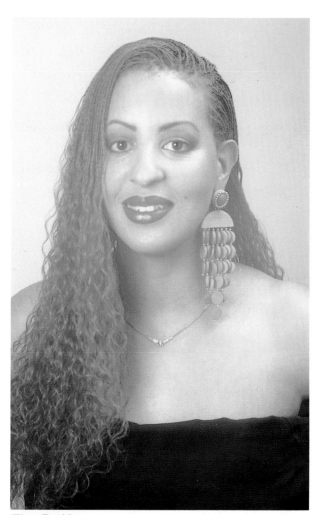

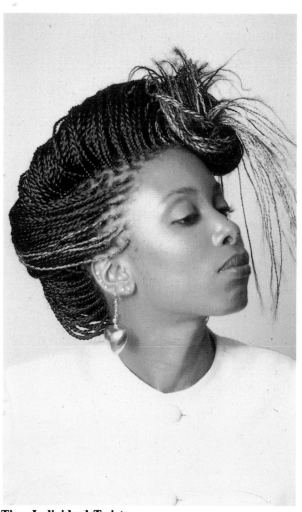

Tiny Braids.
Hairstyle by Carla Brown.

Tiny Individual Twists.
Hairstyle by Carla Brown.

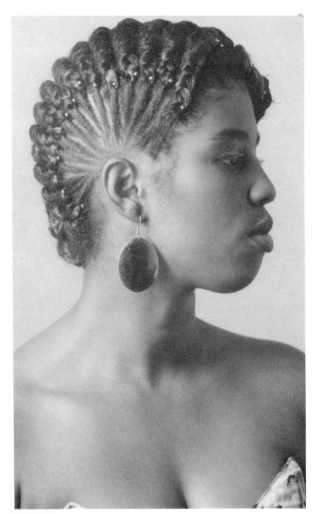 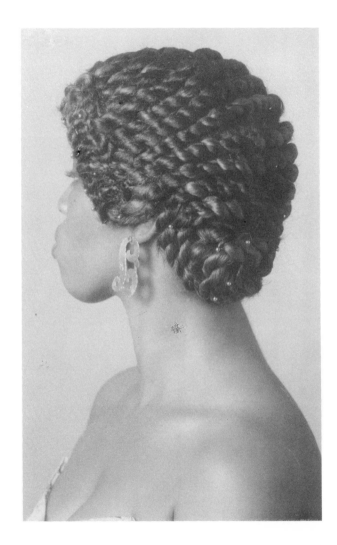

Flat Twists. *Hairstyle by Carla Brown.*

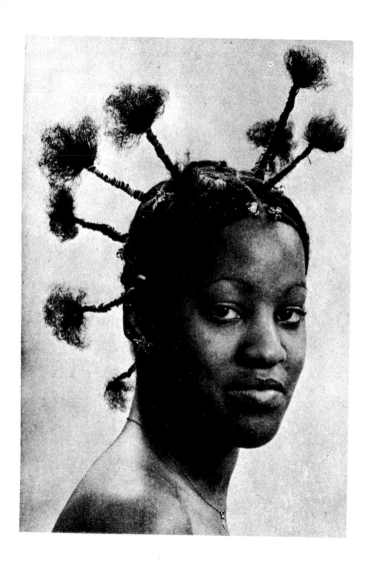

Nakpangi *by Sonia Bullock*

Hair wrapping is common place in West and Central Africa. It is considered suitable for all occassions and all types of dress. Hairwrapping is usually done after the hair has been cornrowed.

All you really need in order to wrap your hair is a comb, brush, bobby pins, rubber bands, thread, wire, and a long-thick head of hair. For best results, the thread should be four strands thick.

The hair wrapping style (pictured) is called Nakpangi. Begin styling Nakpangi by sectioning off the hair into 11 sections. Tie these off with rubber bands.

Hold the hair and thread in your hand. Pull tightly. Beginning at the base of the hair, wrap the thread tightly around the hair. Continue to wrap until you reach the end and then tie the ends of the thread.

When this is completed, the hair may be twisted or shaped in any style desired.

Repeat this same procedure on the other sections.

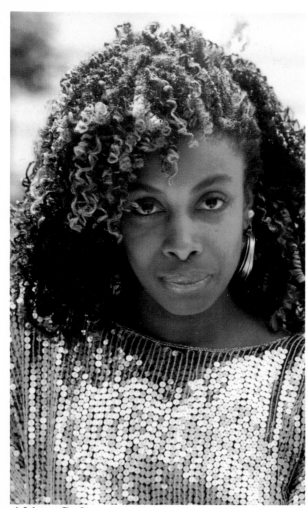

African Curls.
Hairstyle by Carla Brown.

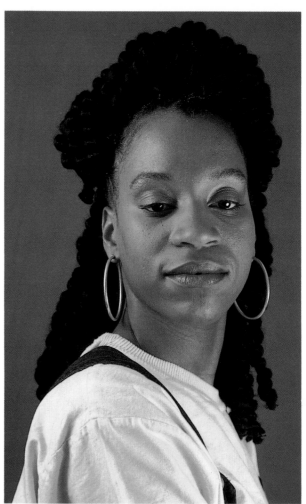

Corkscrews.
Hairstyle by Carla Brown.

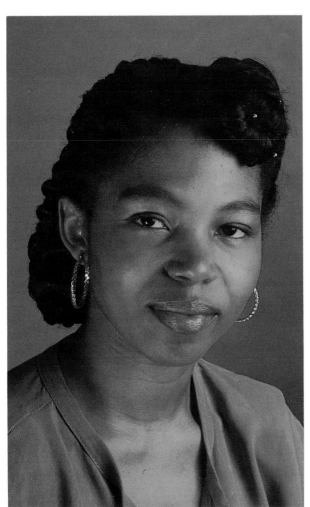
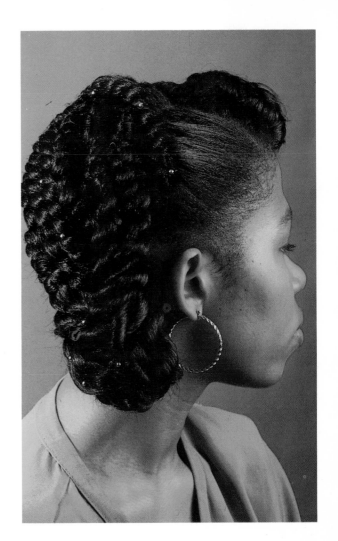

Flat Twists.
Hairstyle by Carla Brown.

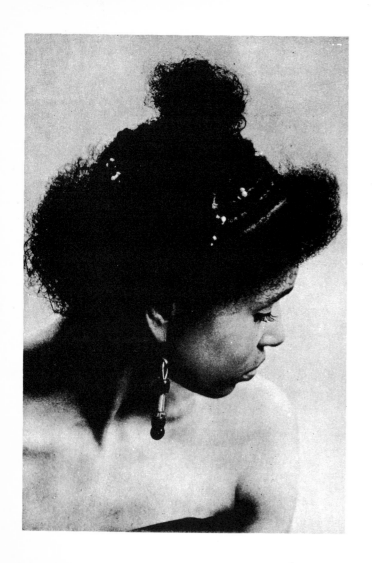

Bush-n-Braid *by Sonia Bullock*

For women who prefer a basic full headed natural, the traditional style of Central Africa's Bushmen gives us the Bush-n-Braid.

This style complements any length or texture of hair. Likewise it can be worn with any style of clothing, day or evening. Styling is as simple as 1-2-3.

Before styling make certain there is a comb, brush, pick, rubber bands, and your choice of adornments available. Adornments are essential to the overall appearance of the Bush-n-Braid, and, as such, should be worn delicately and with care. You might want to try tiny beads, colored pins, or rubber bands.

The best results are achieved when the hair is medium-to-short (although this is not a requirement). The hair should be parted into sections with rubber bands. The number of sections is unimportant. Begin cornrowing around the edges of the hair, back to the center. Then pick out the hair and shape with your hands.

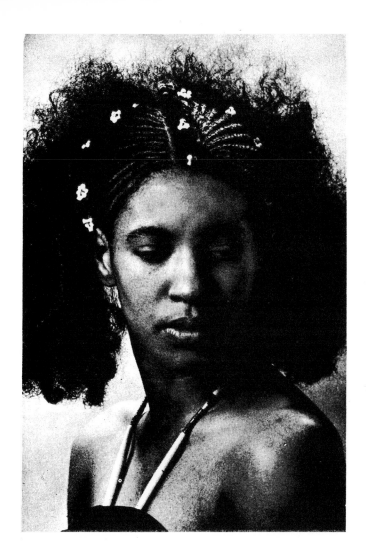

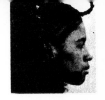

Oshun *by Sonia Bullock*

The Oshun is also inspired by the Bushmen. This simple style also suits all occasions. For most successful appearance, the hair should be thick and medium-to-long in length.

Use the same grooming aides here as in the Bush-n-Braid, adding only rollers to the list.

Now you're ready to style. Begin with one large part from the top of the head. Rubber band the left side and work only on the right. Using this part as a starting point, braid one large braid straight to the front.

Part the hair in half from ear to ear across the top of the head. Section off the back and the left side. Starting at the peak of the forehead, cornrow toward the ear, along the hairline. (Be sure to leave the ends loose.) Continue until the whole head is cornrowed into the center braid. Now take the rubber bands out of left side and repeat these steps.

The back is parted half way up the center, from the neck up. Cornrow from the top of this part to the top of the head. (This should be all one cornrow.) Continue to cornrow all the way around, from part to side of head.

Finally, comb out the ends of the cornrows and curl them with rollers; then pat into shape.

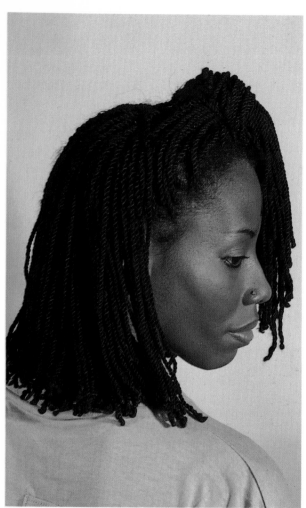

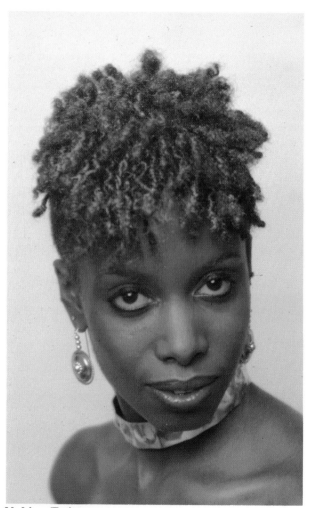

Senegalese Twists.
Hairstyle by Carla Brown.

Nubian Twists.
Hairstyle by Carla Brown.

40

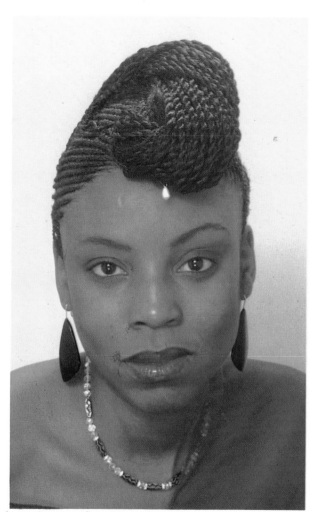

Individual and Cornrow Twists.
Hairstyle by Carla Brown.

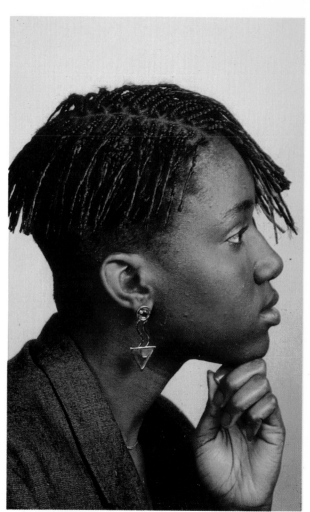

Extension Locs.
Hairstyle by Carla Brown.

41

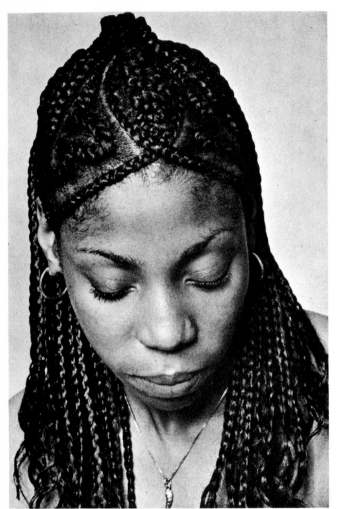

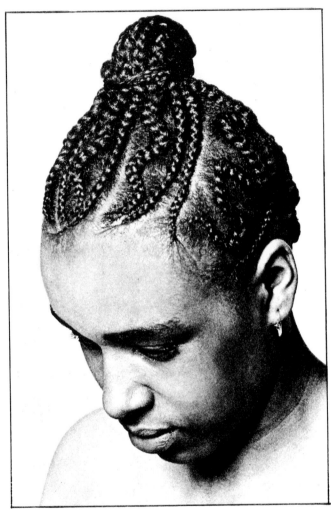

Hairstyles by Donna Moses

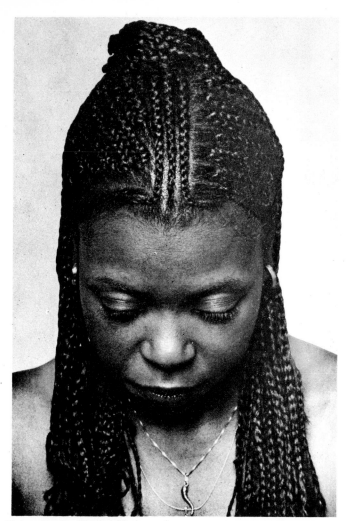

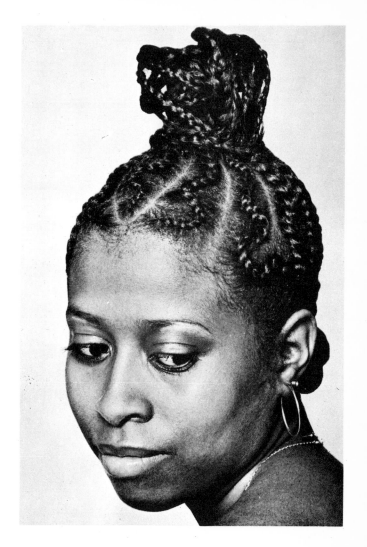

Hairstyles by Donna Moses

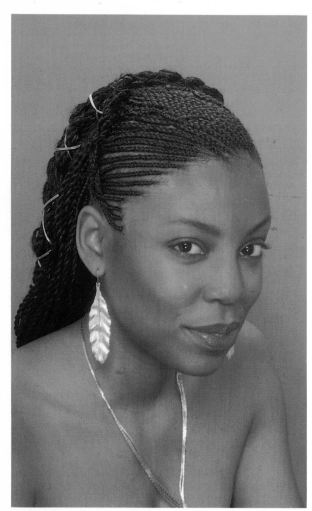

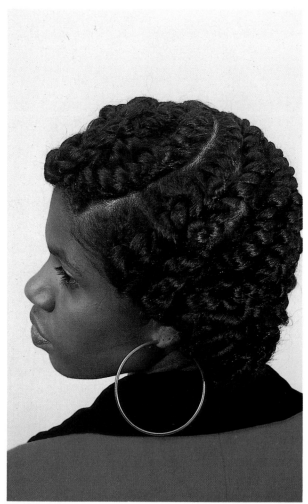

Individual Cornrow Twists.
Hairstyle by Carla Brown.

Flat Twists.
Hairstyle by Carla Brown.

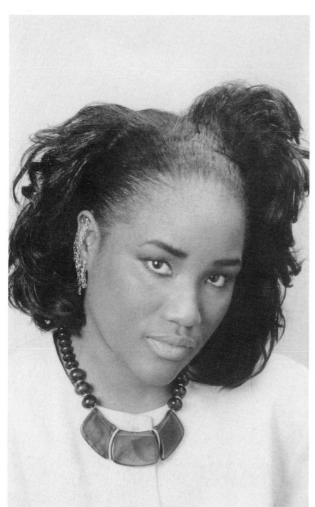

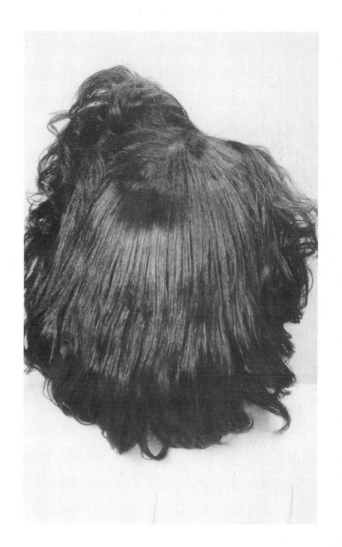

Weave, Cornrow Based.
Hairstyle by Carla Brown.

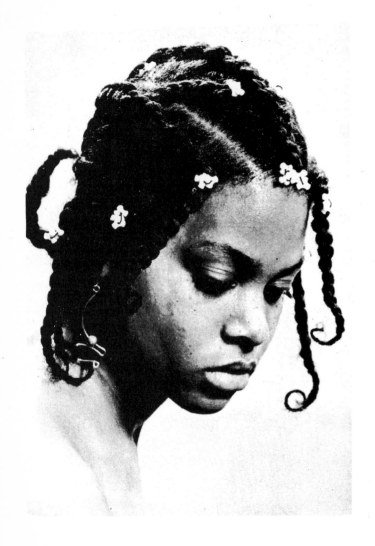

Makeda *by Sonia Bullock*

From ancient Egypt, land of great Black pharaohs and majestic pyramids comes two contemporary styles for Black women with long straight or natural hair. The first of the two the Makeda works best on hair of average thickness, excessively coarse or thick hair will not make for the best results.

The Makeda is an everyday style. It works well with casual attire, but can be dressed up for formal wear.

Before styling hair make sure that rubber bands, bobby pins, small rollers and a comb & brush are nearby.

To begin, part hair in middle. Start with vertical braid; braid a few inches from middle.

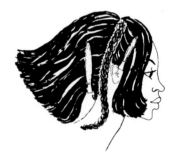

Then braid second vertical braid.

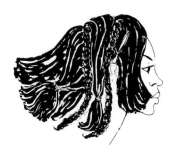

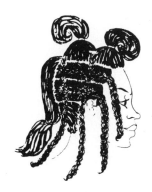

Now, section off remaining hair and begin horizontal braids. Repeat the above steps on the other side of the head.

Now braid center cornrow, making sure that it covers beginnings of all other braids.

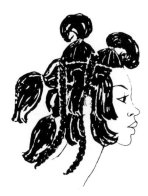

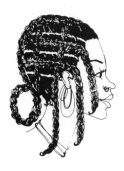

Now you have four braids (or 8 including the other side) crossing over (tic-tac-toe).

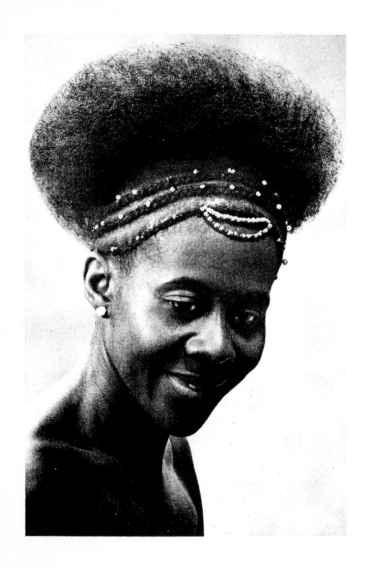

Queen Mother *by Sonia Bullock*

For older and more sedate Black women, there are two hairstyles based on a traditional Ethiopian style: Queen Mother and Wisdom's Crown.

This traditional hairstyle is merely a circular crown of hair, which does not have to be long. The cornrowing is done off the face, around the head. It does not require adornment, but may include a comb or a decorator hair net. Essentially, it is most lovely when worn plain.

Before beginning to create the Queen Mother be sure these are available: rubber bands or barretts, a comb, a brush and a pick.

To begin the Queen Mother, part hair at the lower part of the head and tie the rest with rubber bands or clip with barretts. Begin cornrowing from the back, making certain that each is a complete circle. Repeat this action by gradually removing hair from bands or barretts and making additional cornrows. For medium length, this step should be repeated two more times. Remove the remaining hair from bands or barretts and begin to comb with a pick. Shape this hair with your hands and pat into desired shape. This style is usually worn off the head and should not be perfectly round.

The Queen Mother is most suitable for everyday wear. It can be dressed up by adding beaded hairnets. A simple necklace is most appropriate; earrings, if worn, should be small.

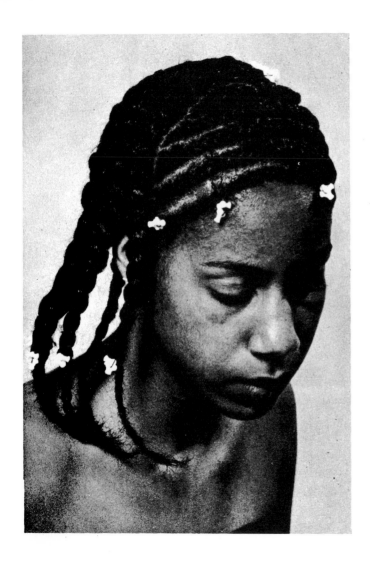

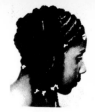

Umoja *by Sonia Bullock*

The second Egyptian inspired style, the Umoja, is designed for the woman with long, thick hair. This style blends with any occasion and any type of dress.

Once again, have a comb, brush, rubber bands, and bobby pins available.

The primary difference between the Makeda and the Umoja is in the sectioning off of the hair. In this case, the hair is parted into 3 sections and this is done for the entire head, not just a half at a time. (The 3 sections should be from temple-to-temple, from behind the ear-to-behind the ear, and the remaining center section.)

Begin by parting the front third of the head, temple to temple, this should be done straight over the top. Now starting on the left side, cornrow four braids across to the right side. Make each of these cornrows about medium in thickness.

Go to the back of head now and cornrow from right to left.

Now concentrate on the center section. Begin here by parting hair for the first cornrow. This cornrow should go left side to right side—connecting these with back braids. Then cornrow across from one ear to the other. Continue now, making two more cornrows. The Fourth and last of these goes in the same direction, except that this one should connect with the front braids, as the first connected with the back.

Ends in front and back can be curled under or allowed to hang loose.

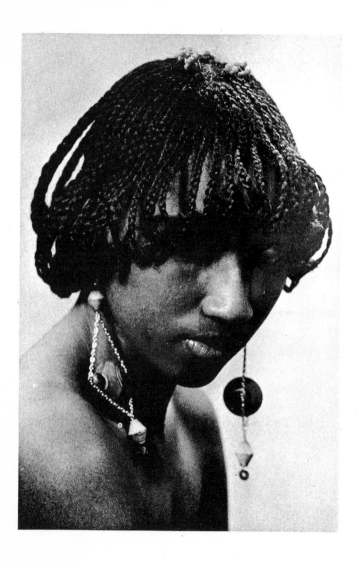

The Bell *by Sonia Bullock*

Black women in Chad, Central Africa, wear their hair in long tight braids, often adorned with cloth or shells. The braiding is done tightly to preserve the natural oils in the scalp from the excessive heat of the sun.

The Bell is worn best by women with thick shoulder length hair. A comb, brush, rubber bands, curlers and hair oil should be available.

Naturally for success with this style or any other, the hair should be washed and conditioned at the outset.

Essentially, the Bell involves sectioning the hair off into 4 sections, with rubber bands. Three of these should be tied off at the beginning.

Concentrating now on only one section, starting at the dome of the head (top) begin cornrowing straight down to the forehead. These rows should be tight, thin cornrows giving the appearance of a twist.

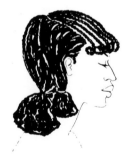

When this is completed, turn your attention to one of

the two side sections. This hair should be parted on a curved slant; this is done to create a rounded effect for the bangs in the front. Begin cornrowing once again—tight, thin cornrows. Repeat this same procedure on the other side of the head.

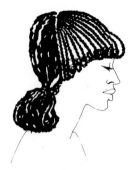

Untie the fourth section of hair. Start just above the ear and part from ear to ear, sectioning off upper portion of hair. Start cornrowing from the sides back to the center of the head.

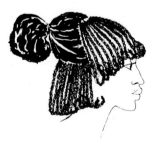

Make these also tight and thin. The shape of these

should be curved. When you reach the center of the head make 2 thin cornrows straight down.

Now repeat this procedure on the upper section. This will complete the back.

By now there should be a group of cornrows hanging at the back of the head. The ends of these cornrows should be rolled with curlers to create desired round or belled effect . . . *Do not use hot curlers,* this will cause breaking off and splitting of hair. Keep the curlers in only long enough for ends to bell.

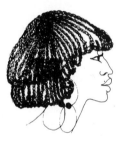

The Bell can be decorated with beads, shells, or flowers. It is most suitable for young women because it involves a great deal of braiding. Although it is essentially a day style, the Bell may be worn in the evening with light adornments. Any neckline is suitable in this case.

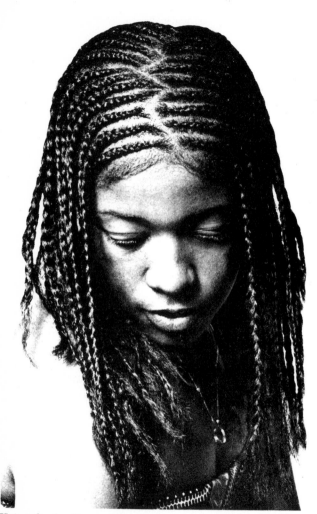

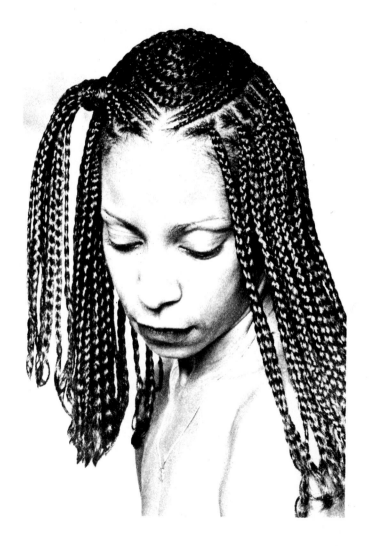

Hairstyles by Donna Moses

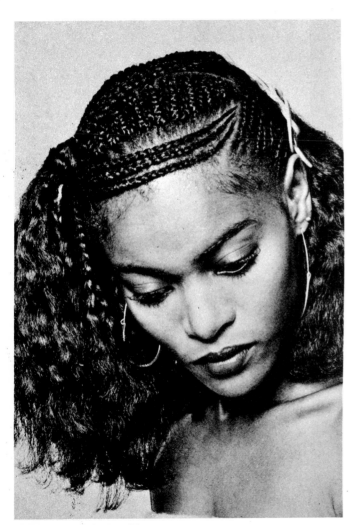

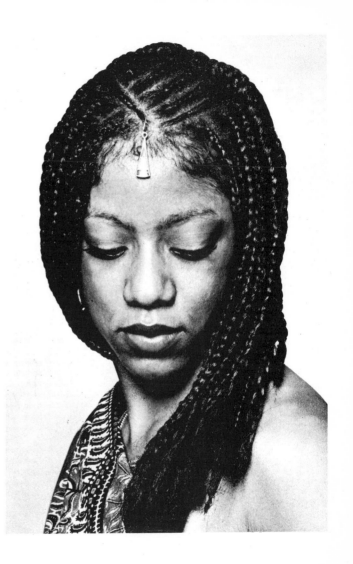

Hairstyles by Donna Moses

53

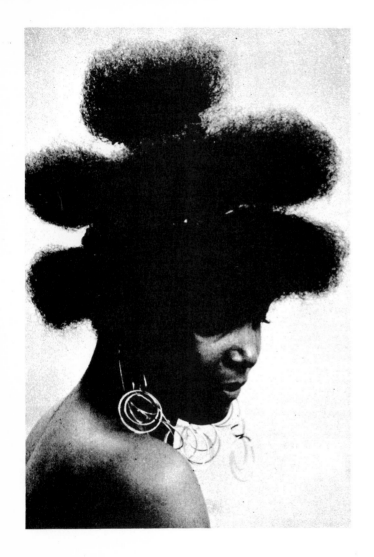

Afro-Pyramid *by Sonia Bullock*

The Afro Pyramid shown here was conceived through the influence of Amenhotep, an early African architect noted for his step-pyramid. Although not exactly a pyramid shape, the traditional style worn in West Africa is essentially an upswept Natural.

This is basically a layered hairstyle for women with long, full, kinky heads of hair. This hair style is most suitable for evening wear. Low necklines and light neck jewelry suit it best.

In preparing to style hair into the Afro-Pyramid, there are some grooming aids necessary: rubber bands, bobby pins and either an Afro puff or hairpiece.

STEP 1 Part your hair and tie it off into 4 sections. (This is done horizontally.)

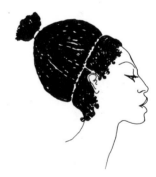

STEP 2 Part the second section and create one thick cornrow along the upper part of section two. By this

time hair should begin to lap over. (Note: all hair should remain sectioned off until all parting within sections and cornrowing is completed.)

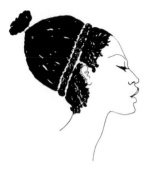

STEP 3 The second layer of the pyramid is created by once again parting the exposed hair, sectioning off, then parting again for a cornrow.

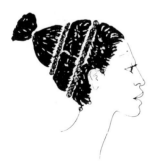

STEP 4 Layer three is actually the top part of the hair, and, at this stage, there is no more parting. With the use of rubber bands, separate the middle of this layer, and add pom poms at the top; this is the fourth layer. If your hair is not long enough to do this, then a hairpiece may be added to create the pom pom effect.

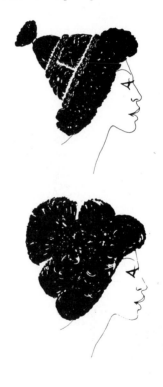

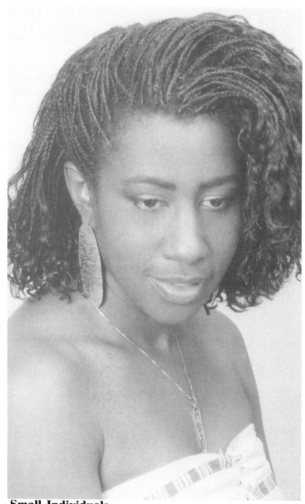

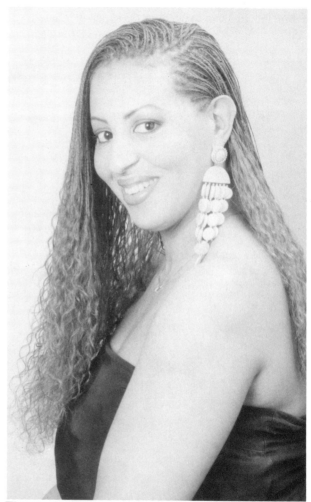

Small Individuals.
Hairstyle by Carla Brown.

Tiny Individuals.
Hairstyle by Carla Brown.

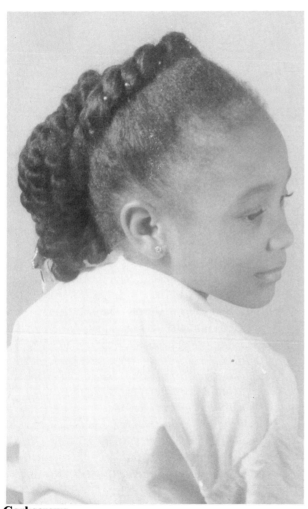
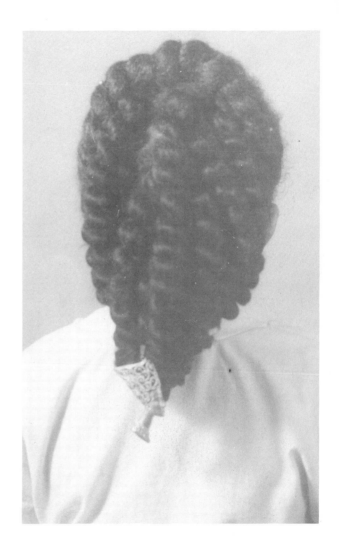

Corkscrews.
Hairstyle by Carla Brown.

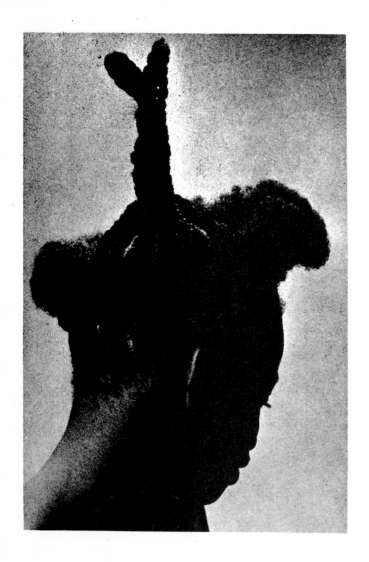

Ayo *by Sonia Bullock*

The Ayo (Joy) is a pleasant style for young girls with long, thick hair. Keep a comb, brush, pick, bobby pins and rubber bands within reach.

Begin by making a part in the circular or lower dome of the head. Take top part and section off 1 section with a rubber band. Next, part hair up the middle to the part at the dome. This should create combed hair on each side of the face. Pin the left side down.

Begin parting on the right side, small tightly pulled braids (up towards the top of the head, away from the face). Please note: the ends should be left loose. Continue this all the way around until you reach the center in back. Take a bobby pin or rubber band out of the other side and do the same thing.

When this is completed, take the rubber band off the top section freeing the hair. With this hair make a 1½ inch part and braid this into a large loose cornrow.

Now, part the hair down the middle and comb it down on the sides, the same as the front. Establish the center of the head; pin one side down and start to part and braid medium size braids up toward the center of the head. Take the remaining braids and wrap them around the base of looped braids and pin.

Starting at the center, connect the smaller front braids by interlocking and then putting in bobby pins all the way around the head to the back. Take out the large cornrow; comb and pick. Pat the hair into shape with your hands.

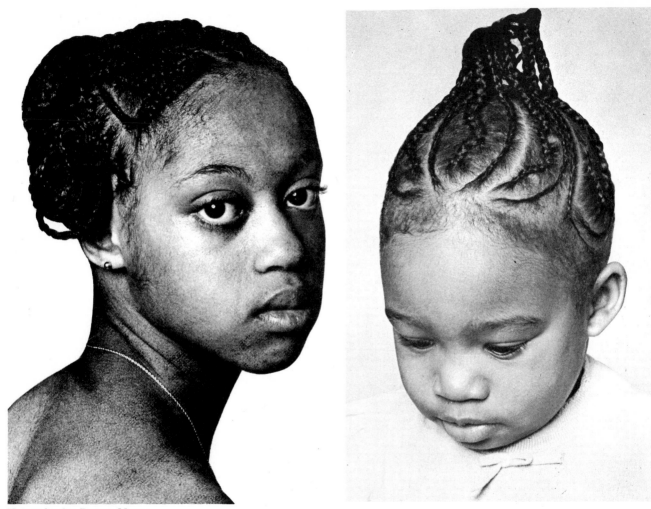

Hairstyles by Donna Moses

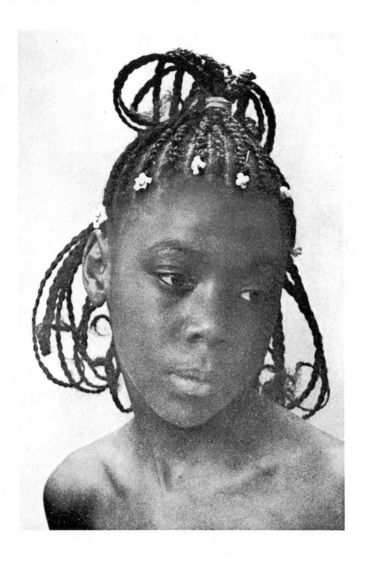

Semi-Bell *by Sonia Bullock*

This second style from Chad is similar to the previous one, except that the hair is not quite as long and the adornments are simpler. From this style, comes today's semi-Bell. As in styling the Bell—use a comb, brush, rubber bands, curlers, barrette and hair oil.

The hair should be parted into 2 sections. The part should be curved from the top of the head down to the temple. Pin down the sides to keep this hair out of the way. Now begin cornrowing from the temple up to the top of the head. These should be small, thin, tight cornrows, as in the Bell. (Make sure that the cornrows are in harmony with the part.) Continue cornrowing all the way around. This should be done on the other side of the curved part as well.

To do the sides, beginning over the ear make a part from behind the ear to the shortest part of the hairline in front. This is done to create a circular effect. Now cornrow and braid 2-3 cornrows and complete this with complementary long, thin braids. Repeat this all along the sides and back. The back should include 4 straight braids down the center of head, the rest is circular. To achieve the rounded effect at the ends use curlers as in the Bell. The top is pulled up with a barrett placed around it.

This style suits younger women, from adolescence up through late teens.

Styling takes about 3 hours.

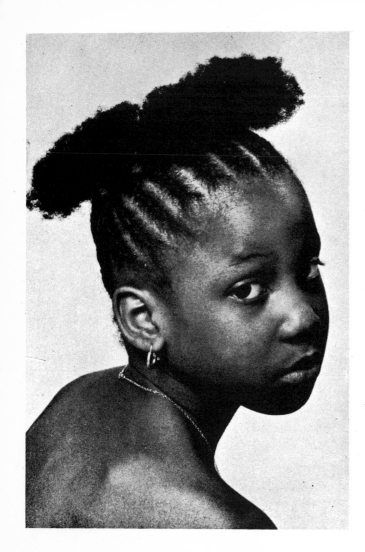

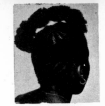

Adeleka *by Sonia Bullock*

The glorification of life as art is present in the Adeleka, a contemporary style similar to the style of Yorubaland women.

Small faced women, with short, kinky hair have the advantage in this case. A comb, brush, pick, rubber bands, and bobby pins are all you need to begin putting "the crown on top".

The first step is to part the hair at the dome of the head, sectioning other hair off. Part down the sides to the ear. Section off the back, creating a front, back and top.

Start cornrowing on the side with medium braids, from hairline to top of the head, all the way around. For the back, start on an angle (photo). Braid from hairline to top of hair (three braids). Part on same angle, but start from top bottom in V shape, continue to other side. On left side, part V shape and braid from left down to center and up to right. Repeat first step—right down, up to left and V shape. So cornrows will be going in different directions, pin down all braids, take top section out and comb out—start at center of head and part outwards, making 8 braids in top of head. Take out pins in front and back and connect these by rubber bands with other braids (see photo). Making 8 braids or puffs, comb out braids, brush and pick—keep rubber bands on. Finally, pat in shape.

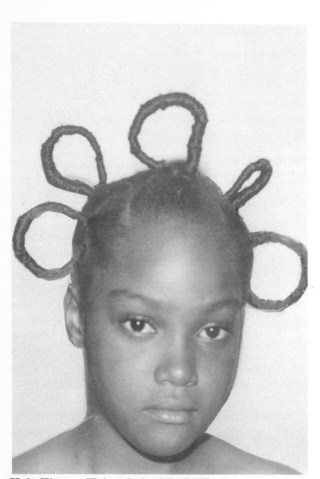
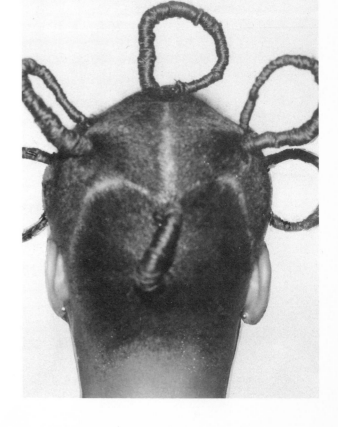

Hair Wraps. *Hairstyle by Nicol Missette.*

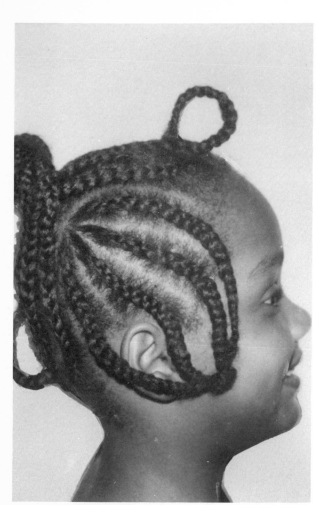
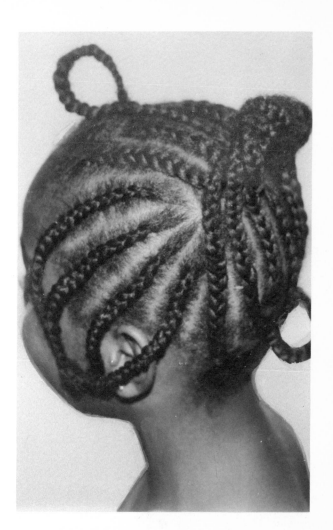

Cornrows. *Hairstyle by Nicol Missette.*

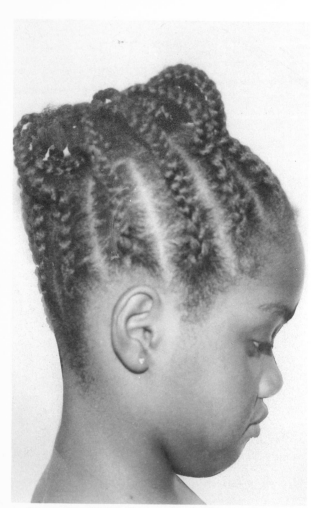

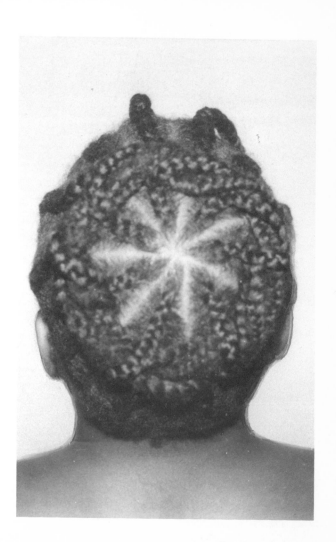

Cornrows. *Hairstyle by Nicol Missette.*

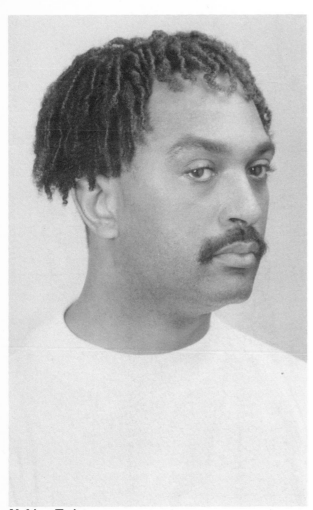

Nubian Twists.
Hairstyle by Carla Brown.

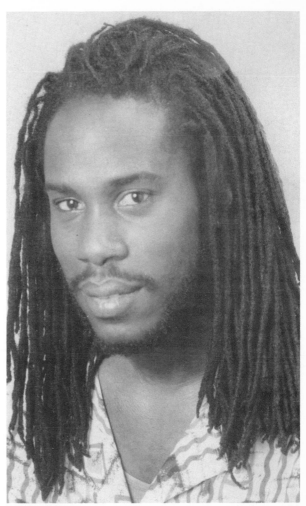

Natural Locs.
Hairstyle by Carla Brown.

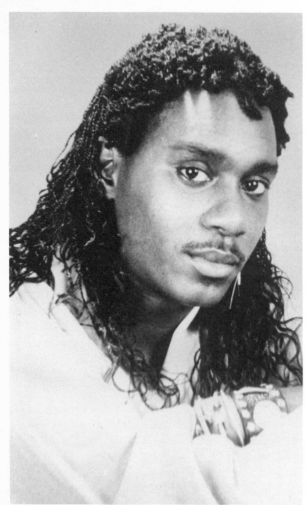

Nubian Twists (front). Individuals (back).
Hairstyle by Carla Brown.

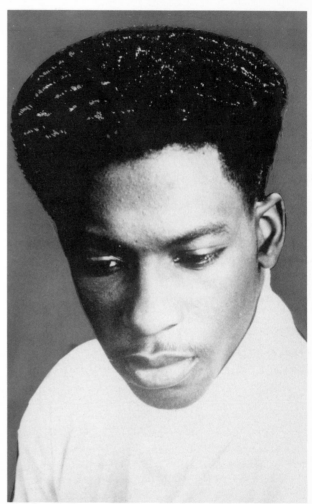

Nubian Twists.
Hairstyle by Carla Brown.

Tips on Hair Grooming.

Care of the Cornrow

When cornrowing, the hair should be wet, already conditioned and lightly toweled. Comb & brush the hair thoroughly and then add oil or conidtioner. Then begin parting and cornrowing. Depending upon the wetness of the hair, a few minutes under the dryer might be advisable.

Care of the Scalp

Cornrowing can be quite healthy for the scalp. Be sure you oil your scalp and hair daily while in cornrows. The cornrows will actually remain in place longer if they are oiled daily and if at night the hair is tied or capped before going to sleep.

A word about Cornrowing and Plaiting

Cornrowing is an underhand motion while plaiting is another name for traditional braiding or pigtailing.

French rolling, which is necessary for styling combination, is merely cornrowing in reverse in an overhand motion.

Sewing Beads into Hair

For sewing you will need thick thread (the same color as the hair). Knot the thread at the end and sew it into the hair, hiding the knot.

Place small beads onto the thread, pushing them all the way down to the end. Now sew again. The entire pattern is then a—"space and sew, space and sew" routine. Do not go all the way to the scalp in sewing, only on top of the cornrow. Repeat this pattern until hair is adorned to your satisfaction.

Beading the Hair

Adorning the hair with beads is easy and adds color and flair to almost any natural or cornrowed style. All you need are small hairpins, bobby pins and, of course, beads.

Just place the hair pin through the hole in the beads. Then slowly stick the beaded hairpin into the hair. Let go of the grip, pushing the hair pin into the hair. Now that the beading is done; make any design you choose.

Note: Beads can be taken out as easily as put in. It is suggested that they be removed before going to bed at night.

Putting Shells into Hair

Shells add a sense of glamor and zest to even the most modest hair style. Shells can be strung on string or thread. In either case this should be thick Chinese style thread. Once the shells are on string or thread, attach them to the hair. Shells can be wrapped into braids or cornrows. Wrap them as if the string or thread were part of the hair. The same procedure can be followed for adorning the hair with bells or rubber bands.